Healing Words
From Heaven

God's Medicine
For Your Health

Healing Words From Heaven
God's Medicine For Your Health

Unless otherwise noted, all Scriptures, and all those marked NKJ, are taken from The New King James Version. Copyright © 1982, Thomas Nelson, Inc. Used by permission.

Scripture marked NIV is from THE HOLY BIBLE: NEW INTERNATIONAL VERSION®. Copyright © 1973,1978,1984 by International Bible Society. Used by permission.

Scripture marked NLT is from the Holy Bible, New Living Translation. Copyright © 1996, Tyndale House Publishers. Used by permission.

Bold emphasis of certain words in Scripture passages is done by the author.

CFA Publications
Box 702032, Tulsa, OK 74170 USA

www.CFApublications.com

Library of Congress Control Number: 2009903411
Library of Congress subject headings:
Spiritual healing — Biblical teaching.
Healing — Biblical teaching.
Healing in the Bible.

ISBN: 978-0-9822097-2-1

He sent forth his word
and healed them;
he rescued them
from the grave.

Psalm 107:20 NIV

Contents

Introduction 7

Healing Is Already Yours 11

Sample Prayer...............................*21*

God's Word Is A Medicine 23

Some Healing Verses 33

Sozo Scriptures 73

Watch Jesus Heal...............................95

Scripture Confessions For Health ...127

Questions...147

Afterword 165

Ordering Information......................167

Introduction

This book will help you receive healing. Jesus Christ paid for it, so healing belongs to you now.

It's written for all who desire to receive God's healing, whether you consider yourself a Christian, or not. Healing is not something you get because you deserve it — it's a free gift from God for all people.

Most of this book is pure Scripture without commentary: many healing verses direct from the Bible in a convenient form. It also includes Scriptures "personalized" for you to confess (say out loud).

This book makes no attempt to teach exhaustively on the subject of healing. Our purpose here is not to cover all the Bible teaches about healing being God's will, but simply to provide some of the healing Scriptures in a concise, easy-to-access format — all that you need to get healed.

We take God at His Word, knowing He cannot lie, and therefore believe that both forgiveness and healing have been provided for all who will believe God's Word and receive them.

There are different ways to receive healing. Thank God for all of them! I am for whatever promotes health, and from what the Bible reveals, I believe God is also.

One way *anyone* can receive healing is to simply believe God's Word and take it as a medicine. This book focuses on this single approach.

Many people think the only way to receive divine healing is to have someone else minister to them. If someone who strongly believes in divine healing does minister to you, it can give you a boost on your road to health. But doing so is like getting a jump-start when your car has a low battery, it may get you going, but to continue running you need to generate your own faith.

It's not wrong to depend on someone else while your faith is growing. But it's a mistake to think you can continue to depend on someone else's faith to get what you need from God forever. God requires us all to grow up and take responsibility for our own lives.

So even if you do receive healing through someone else's faith and ministry, the truths in this book are still vital for you to grasp. In the world we live in, sickness and disease are a constant threat, so your faith needs to be ready. You should not depend on someone else's faith, because they may not always be there when you have a need.

But God's Word is a medicine freely available to all, with the power to make you whole and sound.

Even if doctors have given you a bad report, this book will give you a second opinion — direct from God.

Part of this book was previously published as *Healing Scripture Confessions.* Through the years we have received many testimonies from those who received healing by taking God's medicine. You can be healed in this way, too!

Chapter 1

Healing Is Already Yours

Healing is yours now! Jesus Christ paid a great price to provide healing for you. All you have to do is find out how to receive it.

Healing is available to you now as a free gift from God. You don't have to convince God to heal you. God loves you and has already provided healing for you. It's yours!

You just need to accept healing and receive it, as a gift. You don't have to earn it. Jesus already paid the full price for your healing. (It cost Him His life.)

1 PETER 2:24 NLT
24 He personally carried our
sins in his body on the cross so
that we can be dead to sin and
live for what is right. By his
wounds you are healed.

The Bible is clear: Jesus paid for
mankind's physical healing at the
same time He paid the penalty for
our sins on Calvary.

ISAIAH 53:4-5 NKJ
4 Surely He has borne our
griefs And carried our sorrows;
Yet we esteemed Him stricken,
Smitten by God, and afflicted.
5 But He was wounded for our
transgressions, He was bruised
for our iniquities; The chastisement for our peace was upon
Him, And by His stripes we are
healed.

This passage in Isaiah foretells
the great substitutionary sacrifice

of Jesus Christ on the cross, paying the price to redeem all mankind from the curse resulting from Adam's rebellion. As you can clearly see, it includes healing along with payment for our transgressions.

In Matthew 8 we have the inspired commentary of the Holy Spirit Himself, testifying to the fact that the passage in Isaiah 53:4-5 includes physical healing.

> MATTHEW 8:16-17 NKJ
> 16 When evening had come, they brought to Him many who were demon-possessed. And He cast out the spirits with a word, and healed all who were sick,
> 17 that it might be fulfilled which was spoken by Isaiah the prophet, saying: "He Himself took our infirmities And bore our sicknesses."

For us to receive forgiveness of sins, we must believe Jesus paid the price for our sins. For us to receive healing, we must believe Jesus paid the price for our healing.

Although Jesus has already paid for your healing, He will not force it on you. You still must accept it and possess it. For God will allow whatever you allow in your life.

Many people have been robbed of healing simply because they did not understand that they must actively receive it, instead of waiting on God to do something. They did not realize God has already provided healing for us all through the sacrifice of Jesus at Calvary.

Begging God for something He has already given you is unnecessary. There is no need for you to make promises to God or try to bargain with Him. He has already made provision for your healing, so there is no need to try to get God to do something. Not believing His Word, that He has already given you healing, is really the same as calling God a liar.

Not everyone believes Jesus suffered and died for their sins, just as not everyone believes Jesus suffered and died for their healing.

Those who refuse to believe, cut themselves off from blessings they could enjoy. But *whoever* will believe, no matter how much they have sinned, or how sick they are, can receive forgiveness and healing.

God has already provided for your healing and health, but you must still receive that provision by faith. That means you must believe what

God said. Of course, you must first know what God said, in order to believe what He said. That's why the healing Scriptures are in this book, so you can know the truth.

God is not mad at you. He has forgiven you. He is for you — not against you. It's His will for you to be healed — whoever you are.

God does not withhold healing from anyone. It's the devil who tries to stop it (through ignorance, doubt, unbelief, confusion, and discouragement). But the devil is defeated and must yield to God's Word spoken in faith from the mouth of a believer.

Sickness is your enemy whose purpose is to steal from you and kill you (John 10:10). But you have authority over all sickness through what Jesus Christ did for you.

God loved you so much He sent Jesus as your substitute, suffering and dying in your place, to set you free from the curse, which includes all sickness and disease. Now Jesus Christ is alive, and He is Lord over all, so sickness and disease must yield to the mighty authority of Jesus' Name.

As a believer you have the right to use the authority of Jesus' Name to command every sickness to leave you.

All healing is a process that happens through time as you continually improve in health. With God, healing can sometimes be so speeded up that to us it seems almost instant, but this is not the normal way God's healing works.

Jesus taught us that God's kingdom works like a seed planted in

the ground which grows and pro-
duces over time (Matthew 13:31).

The important thing, and what
God's Word promises, is the end
result, not how long it takes.

Many people who have not understood that healing from God is a
process involving time, have given
up their faith when they did not
have an instant miracle recovery.

Don't let the devil steal from you,
through this wrong thinking, what
Jesus paid for you to have!

The Bible tells us that healing is
ours, because Jesus paid for it. But
the Bible never says we will all receive healing instantly. Sometimes
it can be very quick — and we know
it is a miracle. Other times it can
take awhile, but no matter how
long it takes, we have the promise

of God that healing is ours, giving us divine assurance that we will be healthy and whole!

Yes, healing from God's Word comes in "seed form" which has to be planted in your heart to see its full fruit. But, once planted and watered, God's living Word will bring healing and health to all your flesh.

To heal is to make sound or whole, to restore to health. This is what God does through His Word in our lives and in our bodies when we allow Him, because it is His nature.

This book emphasizes only one of the many ways we can receive God's healing — through His Word. Since God is a healer, everything He made has some healing virtue in it, and therefore God's healing can come to you in many ways.

Nutritious food, clean water, fresh air, and sunshine all promote health. Many sicknesses can be overcome simply by taking in these healthy nutrients God has provided for us. The human body is designed by God to heal itself when we give it what it needs.

But even if you are missing some needed nutrition, God's Word can still bring you healing. The Word that created the human body can bring it healing.

Never forget, or doubt: healing belongs to you now, because Jesus already paid for it, and gave it to you as a free gift!

So don't let the devil steal healing and health from you!

Sample Prayer

Father God, your Word, the Holy Bible, says healing was provided for me through the sacrifice of Jesus Christ. I believe you are not a liar.

So, by faith in what you said in the Bible, I accept your forgiveness and healing now, as a free gift. I know I don't deserve it because of anything I have done, but I thank you for giving it to me because of Jesus.

I say that Jesus Christ is Lord of my life and my body. He rose from death, victorious over satan, sin, and sickness.   >>>

So, all sickness and disease, I command you in the Name of Jesus to leave my body now. Leave me alone, satan! Jesus Christ is now my Lord.

I believe healing and health is mine because of what Jesus did for me, and I receive, as a gift from God, complete healing for my entire body now.

Body of mine, I speak to you and command you in Jesus' Name to be healed, healthy, and whole.

Thank You Lord Jesus that your healing power is working in my body now. Thank You for healing me!

Chapter 2

God's Word Is A Medicine

Medicine is something that treats, prevents, or alleviates the symptoms of disease.

God's Word is a medicine freely available to all. It has power not only to treat symptoms, but also to make people whole and sound. It is effective for all conditions that afflict mankind.

You can take God's Word as a medicine with no danger of an overdose. And you don't have to buy it. It's free to you, because Jesus already paid for it with His life!

But like any medicine, God's Word has to be taken to be effective. Medicine on a shelf never healed anyone. You must take it according to the directions.

Here are the directions:

> PROVERBS 4:20-23 NLT
> 20 My child, pay attention to what I say. Listen carefully to my words.
> 21 Don't lose sight of them. Let them penetrate deep into your heart,
> 22 for they bring life to those who find them, and healing to their whole body.
> 23 Guard your heart above all else, for it determines the course of your life.

Verse 22 tells us that God's words will bring healing to our whole body.

"Medicine" is the word we use today to describe what brings us healing and health when we are sick. So that is why we say that God's written Word can be described as a medicine.

Often doctors prescribe medicine for us to take while we are in the process of healing. God has freely given us His Word to take regularly as His medicine, without charge.

If you will be as diligent to take God's Word as a medicine as you would the doctor's prescription, you will see wonderful results.

God's medicine works by taking His Word into your being. You do that by listening to the Word, reading the Word, speaking the Word, and meditating on it. (Meditating means to think about it, imagine it, and speak it to yourself.)

PSALM 107:20 NKJ
20 He sent His word and
healed them, and delivered
them from their destructions.

God's Word will produce what God
sent it to do: healing and health.
It functions as a seed to produce
a harvest of blessing in your life, if
you keep it in your heart.

LUKE 8:11 NKJ
11 "Now the parable is this:
The seed is the word of God.

God's Word is alive. Just like a
seed — the words of the Bible are
full of unseen life.

JOHN 6:63 NKJ
63 "It is the Spirit who gives
life; the flesh profits nothing.
The words that I speak to you
are spirit, and they are life.

HEBREWS 4:12a NLT
12 For the word of God is alive
and powerful.

God's written Word has a super-
natural quality which imparts life
to us. Just because we cannot feel
the healing power coming from
God's Word proves nothing.

People can be in the presence of
deadly atomic radiation without
feeling anything, but it still causes
harmful change to take place in
their bodies.

God's Words recorded in the Bible
may seem dead and lifeless, just
as seeds do. But they are alive and
impart life and health to our whole
body.

JOHN 8:31-32 NKJ
31 Then Jesus said to those
Jews who believed Him, "If you

abide in My word, you are My
disciples indeed.
32 "And you shall know the
truth, and the truth shall make
you free."

You have the written guarantee
of Jesus — His Word will produce
freedom, including freedom from
sickness. But, you must abide, or
continue in His Word. You must
feed on God's Word until you know
that you know the truth. Then you
will act on that truth — and it will
make you free.

Taking God's Word as our medicine involves listening to, and believing, what God said. We must
put what God says above what
anyone else may say. No one has
higher authority, knowledge, or
ability than God. So we can trust
what God says above what anyone
else says.

Whenever we start to meditate on our symptoms of sickness and negative reports, which is called "worry," we have quit taking God's Word as a medicine in accordance with the directions given in the Bible.

Worry is the wrong focus, meditating on the wrong thing. Bible meditation involves your imagination. It also includes what you think about, and what you say to yourself, inwardly as well as vocally.

How do you see yourself? Do you see yourself getting well? Or do you see yourself getting worse? If you are correctly meditating on God's Words, you will "see yourself" getting better. You will think, talk, and act in line with getting well.

Words are how we communicate our decisions and our faith: to ourselves, to God, to the devil, and to other people. When we decide to believe God's Word (that healing is ours), we will begin to speak accordingly.

The Bible tells us to "hold fast" to speaking in agreement with God's Word (Hebrews 4:14, 10:23) — because there is always a spiritual struggle trying to get us to quit.

So "Hang on tight!" Keep on believing and speaking your faith! Fight the good fight of faith! You will have to resist the temptation to doubt. But regardless of your symptoms or feelings, healing belongs to you, so don't let the devil steal it from you by doubting God's Word.

We must choose to look beyond our temporary physical symptoms to the eternal written Word of Almighty God — Who cannot lie.

It is a mistake to base our beliefs only on something as unreliable as our physical senses. But we can depend on God's Word.

Remember that God's Word works as a medicine in your body, bringing you health and wholeness, while you focus your attention on God's Word by keeping it in your heart, mind, and mouth.

God's Word will certainly heal. It is full of God's power and carries the authority of God who spoke it. We just have to "hang on" to God's Word and let it do its work.

Whatever sickness or disease you suffer from, God's Word will cure it. All we see was created by God speaking words. Because God used His Words to create, His Words can also bring healing to what He created.

PROVERBS 4:22 NLT
22 for they bring life to those who find them, and healing to their whole body.

If you faithfully take God's Word, you'll find it's the best medicine. Make sure you take it diligently until you see yourself as God's Word says you are.

Even if satisfactory results are not obtained right away just persevere because you can't overdose on God's medicine. In fact, the more of God's medicine you take, the better off you will be!

God's Word is the perfect medicine. There are no bad side effects, it works on every illness, and everyone can afford it.

Chapter 3

Some Healing Verses

This chapter contains verses for your meditation. From the New King James translation, they are large to make them easy to read, and to emphasize their importance.

Those not specifically about healing are about faith, which is how we receive healing.

Feast long and often on each verse, for they are truly full of life. These words from God contain the same kind of life in them that God used when He created mankind with His Word.

"I am the LORD who heals you."

Exodus 15:26b

"So you shall serve
the LORD your God,
and He will bless
your bread and your
water. And I will take
sickness away from the
midst of you.

Exodus 23:25

"No one shall suffer miscarriage or be barren in your land; I will fulfill the number of your days.

Exodus 23:26

"God is not a man, that He should lie, Nor a son of man, that He should repent. Has He said, and will He not do? Or has He spoken, and will He not make it good?

Numbers 23:19

"And the LORD will take away from you all sickness,

Deuteronomy 7:15a

I have set before
you life and death,
blessing and cursing;
therefore choose life,
that both you and your
descendants may live;

Deuteronomy 30:19b

With long life I will
satisfy him, And show
him My salvation."

Psalm 91:16

Bless the LORD, O
my soul, And forget
not all His benefits:
Who forgives all your
iniquities, Who heals
all your diseases,

Psalm 103:2-3

He sent His word and
healed them, And
delivered them from
their destructions.

Psalm 107:20

I shall not die, but live,
And declare the works
of the LORD.

Psalm 118:17

My son, give attention to my words; Incline your ear to my sayings. Do not let them depart from your eyes; Keep them in the midst of your heart; For they are life to those who find them, And health to all their flesh.

Proverbs 4:20-22

Fear not, for I am with you; Be not dismayed, for I am your God. I will strengthen you, Yes, I will help you, I will uphold you with My righteous right hand.'

Isaiah 41:10

But He was wounded
for our transgressions,
He was bruised for
our iniquities; The
chastisement for our
peace was upon Him,
And by His stripes we
are healed.

Isaiah 53:5

For I know the thoughts that I think toward you, says the LORD, thoughts of peace and not of evil, to give you a future and a hope.

Jeremiah 29:11

And Jesus went about
all Galilee, teaching
in their synagogues,
preaching the gospel
of the kingdom, and
healing all kinds of
sickness and all kinds
of disease among the
people.

Matthew 4:23

Your kingdom come.
Your will be done
On earth as it is in
heaven.

Matthew 6:10

When evening had
come, they brought to
Him many who were
demon-possessed.
And He cast out the
spirits with a word,
and healed all who
were sick, that it might
be fulfilled which
was spoken by Isaiah
the prophet, saying:
"He Himself took our
infirmities And bore
our sicknesses."

Matthew 8:16-17

"What do you mean, 'If I can'?" Jesus asked. "Anything is possible if a person believes."

Mark 9:23

"For assuredly, I say
to you, whoever says
to this mountain, 'Be
removed and be cast
into the sea,' and does
not doubt in his heart,
but believes that those
things he says will
be done, he will have
whatever he says.

Mark 11:23

"Therefore I say to you, whatever things you ask when you pray, believe that you receive them, and you will have them.

And whenever you stand praying, if you have anything against anyone, forgive him, that your Father in heaven may also forgive you your trespasses.

Mark 11:24-25

But when Jesus heard it, He answered him, saying, "Do not be afraid; only believe, and she will be made well."

Luke 8:50

He sent them to preach
the kingdom of God
and to heal the sick.

Luke 9:2

"So ought not this woman, being a daughter of Abraham, whom Satan has bound — think of it — for eighteen years, be loosed from this bond on the Sabbath?"

Luke 13:16

"If you abide in My word, you are My disciples indeed. "And you shall know the truth, and the truth shall make you free."

John 8:31b-32

Also a multitude
gathered from the
surrounding cities to
Jerusalem, bringing
sick people and those
who were tormented
by unclean spirits, and
they were all healed.

Acts 5:16

But if the Spirit of Him who raised Jesus from the dead dwells in you, He who raised Christ from the dead will also give life to your mortal bodies through His Spirit who dwells in you.

Romans 8:11

And since we have the same spirit of faith, according to what is written, "I believed and therefore I spoke," we also believe and therefore speak,

2 Corinthians 4:13

while we do not look
at the things which
are seen, but at the
things which are not
seen. For the things
which are seen are
temporary, but the
things which are not
seen are eternal.

2 Corinthians 4:18

casting down
arguments and every
high thing that exalts
itself against the
knowledge of God,
bringing every thought
into captivity to the
obedience of Christ,

2 Corinthians 10:5

Christ has redeemed us from the curse of the law, having become a curse for us (for it is written, "Cursed is everyone who hangs on a tree"), that the blessing of Abraham might come upon the Gentiles in Christ Jesus, that we might receive the promise of the Spirit through faith.

Galatians 3:13,14

above all, taking the
shield of faith with
which you will be able
to quench all the fiery
darts of the wicked
one.

Ephesians 6:16

for it is God who works
in you both to will
and to do for His good
pleasure.

Philippians 2:13

Now may the God of
peace Himself sanctify
you completely; and
may your whole spirit,
soul, and body be
preserved blameless at
the coming of our Lord
Jesus Christ.

1 Thessalonians 5:23

Fight the good fight of faith, lay hold on eternal life, to which you were also called and have confessed the good confession in the presence of many witnesses.

1 Timothy 6:12

For God has not given
us a spirit of fear, but
of power and of love
and of a sound mind.

2 Timothy 1:7

Now faith is the
substance of things
hoped for, the evidence
of things not seen.

Hebrews 11:1

And the prayer of faith
will save the sick, and
the Lord will raise
him up. And if he has
committed sins, he will
be forgiven.

James 5:15

who Himself bore
our sins in His own
body on the tree, that
we, having died to
sins, might live for
righteousness — by
whose stripes you were
healed.

1 Peter 2:24

Beloved, I pray that
you may prosper in
all things and be in
health, just as your
soul prospers.

3 John 1:2

Chapter 4

Sozo Scriptures

The New Testament was written in Greek, so all English versions are translations. Some words have more than one meaning, so translators have to choose which word they think is best. Obviously their beliefs affect how they translate.

The New Testament Greek word "sozo" is usually translated "save" but its meaning includes deliverance from all danger and suffering. It means to make whole, safe, sound, and well; to heal and restore to health.

Being "saved" is not limited to being born again. It also includes healing. It means total deliverance.

The following verses show how the translators realize that "sozo" could also refer to physical healing. The bold words are the English translation of the Greek word "sozo."

MARK 5:23 NKJ
23 and begged Him earnestly, saying, "My little daughter lies at the point of death. Come and lay Your hands on her, that she may **be healed**, and she will live."

MARK 10:52 NKJ
52 Then Jesus said to him, "Go your way; your faith has **made you well**." And immediately he received his sight and followed Jesus on the road.

LUKE 8:36 NKJ
36 They also who had seen it told them by what means he who had been demon-possessed **was healed**.

LUKE 18:42 NKJ
42 Then Jesus said to him, "Receive your sight; your faith has **made you well**."

ACTS 14:9 NKJ
9 This man heard Paul speaking. Paul, observing him intently and seeing that he had faith to **be healed**,

The following seventeen verses, in large print, are from the New King James translation, except for the words in bold, which have been changed to reflect what we have discovered about the meaning of the word "sozo."

Based on the meaning of the New Testament Greek word "sozo," the words "save" and "saved" have been changed in the following verses to "heal" and "healed," for you to meditate on.

Although the NKJ translators did not choose to use the words in bold, they surely could have without distorting the meaning the original hearers of Scripture understood. Because, as we have seen, the meaning of "sozo" clearly includes deliverance from physical sickness.

The true meaning of these verses is not limited to physical healing, but certainly includes physical healing. Faith works the same for receiving healing as it does for receiving forgiveness of sins and the new birth.

"Those by the wayside are the ones who hear; then the devil comes and takes away the word out of their hearts, lest they should believe and be **healed**.

Luke 8:12

"For the Son of Man did not come to destroy men's lives but to **heal** them."

Luke 9:56a

"for the Son of Man has come to seek and to **heal** that which was lost."

Luke 19:10

"For God did not send His Son into the world to condemn the world, but that the world through Him might be **healed**.

John 3:17

"And if anyone hears My words and does not believe, I do not judge him; for I did not come to judge the world but to **heal** the world.

John 12:47

"Nor is there salvation in any other, for there is no other name under heaven given among men by which we must be **healed**."

Acts 4:12

'who will tell you words by which you and all your household will be **healed**.'

Acts 11:14

"But we believe that through the grace of the Lord Jesus Christ we shall be **healed** in the same manner as they."

Acts 15:11

So they said, "Believe on the Lord Jesus Christ, and you will be **healed**, you and your household."

Acts 16:31

that if you confess with
your mouth the Lord
Jesus and believe in
your heart that God
has raised Him from
the dead, you will be
healed.

Romans 10:9

For "whoever calls on the name of the LORD shall be **healed**."

Romans 10:13

For since, in the wisdom of God, the world through wisdom did not know God, it pleased God through the foolishness of the message preached to **heal** those who believe.

1 Corinthians 1:21

For by grace you have been **healed** through faith, and that not of yourselves; it is the gift of God,

Ephesians 2:8

This is a faithful saying and worthy of all acceptance, that Christ Jesus came into the world to **heal** sinners, of whom I am chief.

1 Timothy 1:15

For this is good and acceptable in the sight of God our Savior, who desires all men to be **healed** and to come to the knowledge of the truth.

1 Timothy 2:3-4

Therefore He is also
able to **heal** to the
uttermost those
who come to God
through Him, since He
always lives to make
intercession for them.

Hebrews 7:25

And the prayer of faith will **heal** the sick, and the Lord will raise him up. And if he has committed sins, he will be forgiven.

James 5:15

Chapter 5

Watch Jesus Heal

As you read the healing accounts on the following pages, never forget that Jesus demonstrated God's will for us in all He did, and He is still the same today (Hebrews 13:8).

Also after Jesus went to Heaven, He continued to do the same works of healing through His disciples.

> ACTS 10:38 NKJ
> 38 "how God anointed Jesus of Nazareth with the Holy Spirit and with power, who went about doing good and healing all who were oppressed by the devil, for God was with Him."

MATTHEW 4:23-24 NKJ
23 Now Jesus went about
all Galilee, teaching in their
synagogues, preaching the
gospel of the kingdom, and
healing all kinds of sickness
and all kinds of disease
among the people.
24 Then His fame went
throughout all Syria; and
they brought to Him all sick
people who were afflicted
with various diseases and
torments, and those who
were demon-possessed, epi-
leptics, and paralytics; and
He healed them.

MATTHEW 8:7-8,13 NKJ
7 And Jesus said to him, "I will come and heal him."
8 The centurion answered and said, "Lord, I am not worthy that You should come under my roof. But only speak a word, and my servant will be healed."
13 Then Jesus said to the centurion, "Go your way; and as you have believed, so let it be done for you." And his servant was healed that same hour.

MATTHEW 8:15-17 NKJ
15 And He touched her
hand, and the fever left her.
Then she arose and served
them.
16 When evening had come,
they brought to Him many
who were demon-possessed.
And He cast out the spirits
with a word, and healed all
who were sick,
17 that it might be fulfilled
which was spoken by Isaiah
the prophet, saying: "He
Himself took our infirmities
and bore our sicknesses."

MATTHEW 9:35 NKJ

35 And Jesus went about all the cities and villages, teaching in their synagogues, preaching the gospel of the kingdom, and healing every sickness and every disease among the people.

MATTHEW 12:10,13 NKJ
10 And behold, there was
a man who had a withered
hand. And they asked Him,
saying, "Is it lawful to heal
on the Sabbath?" — that
they might accuse Him.
13 Then He said to the man,
"Stretch out your hand."
And he stretched it out, and
it was restored as whole as
the other.

MATTHEW 12:15 NKJ
15 But when Jesus knew it, He withdrew from there; and great multitudes followed Him, and He healed them all.

MATTHEW 12:22 NKJ

22 Then one was brought to Him who was demon-possessed, blind and mute; and He healed him, so that the blind and mute man both spoke and saw.

MATTHEW 13:15 NKJ
15 for the heart of this people has grown dull. Their ears are hard of hearing, and their eyes they have closed, lest they should see with their eyes and hear with their ears, lest they should understand with their heart and turn, so that I should heal them.

MATTHEW 14:14 NKJ
14 And when Jesus went out He saw a great multitude; and He was moved with compassion for them, and healed their sick.

MATTHEW 15:28 NKJ
28 Then Jesus answered
and said to her, "O woman,
great is your faith! Let it be
to you as you desire." And
her daughter was healed
from that very hour.

MATTHEW 15:30 NKJ
30 Then great multitudes
came to Him, having with
them those who were lame,
blind, mute, maimed, and
many others; and they laid
them down at Jesus' feet,
and He healed them.

MATTHEW 17:18 NKJ
18 And Jesus rebuked the demon, and it came out of him; and the child was cured from that very hour.

MATTHEW 19:2 NKJ
2 And great multitudes followed Him, and He healed
them there.

MATTHEW 21:14 NKJ
14 Then the blind and the lame came to Him in the temple, and He healed them.

MARK 1:34 NKJ

34 Then He healed many who were sick with various diseases, and cast out many demons; and He did not allow the demons to speak, because they knew Him.

MARK 3:10 NKJ
10 For He healed many, so that as many as had afflictions pressed about Him to touch Him.

MARK 6:5-6 NKJ

5 Now He could do no mighty work there, except that He laid His hands on a few sick people and healed them.

6 And He marveled because of their unbelief. Then He went about the villages in a circuit, teaching.

LUKE 4:18 NKJ

18 "The Spirit of the Lord is upon Me, because He has anointed Me to preach the gospel to the poor. He has sent Me to heal the broken-hearted, to preach deliverance to the captives and recovery of sight to the blind, to set at liberty those who are oppressed,"

LUKE 4:40 NKJ

40 Now when the sun was setting, all those who had anyone sick with various diseases brought them to Him; and He laid His hands on every one of them and healed them.

LUKE 5:15 NKJ
15 Then the report went around concerning Him all the more; and great multitudes came together to hear, and to be healed by Him of their infirmities.

LUKE 6:17-19 NKJ

17 And He came down with them and stood on a level place with a crowd of His disciples and a great multitude of people from all Judea and Jerusalem, and from the seacoast of Tyre and Sidon, who came to hear Him and be healed of their diseases,

18 as well as those who were tormented with unclean spirits. And they were healed.

19 And the whole multitude sought to touch Him, for power went out from Him and healed them all.

LUKE 8:43-44 NKJ
43 Now a woman, having a flow of blood for twelve years, who had spent all her livelihood on physicians and could not be healed by any, 44 came from behind and touched the border of His garment. And immediately her flow of blood stopped.

LUKE 8:47-48 NKJ

47 Now when the woman saw that she was not hidden, she came trembling; and falling down before Him, she declared to Him in the presence of all the people the reason she had touched Him and how she was healed immediately.

48 And He said to her, "Daughter, be of good cheer; your faith has made you well. Go in peace."

LUKE 9:11 NKJ
11 But when the multi-
tudes knew it, they followed
Him; and He received them
and spoke to them about
the kingdom of God, and
healed those who had need
of healing.

LUKE 13:11-16 NKJ

11 And behold, there was a woman who had a spirit of infirmity eighteen years, and was bent over and could in no way raise herself up.

12 But when Jesus saw her, He called her to Him and said to her, "Woman, you are loosed from your infirmity."

13 And He laid His hands on her, and immediately she was made straight, and glorified God.

14 But the ruler of the synagogue answered with indignation, because Jesus had healed on the Sabbath; and he said to the crowd, "There are six days on which men ought to work; therefore come and be healed on them, and not on the Sabbath day."

15 The Lord then answered him and said . . .

16 "So ought not this woman, being a daughter of Abraham, whom Satan has bound —think of it — for eighteen years, be loosed from this bond on the Sabbath?"

LUKE 14:3-4 NKJ

3 And Jesus, answering, spoke to the lawyers and Pharisees, saying, "Is it lawful to heal on the Sabbath?" 4 But they kept silent. And He took him and healed him, and let him go.

LUKE 17:12-15 NKJ

12 Then as He entered a certain village, there met Him ten men who were lepers, who stood afar off.

13 And they lifted up their voices and said, "Jesus, Master, have mercy on us!"

14 So when He saw them, He said to them, "Go, show yourselves to the priests." And so it was that as they went, they were cleansed.

15 Now one of them, when he saw that he was healed, returned, and with a loud voice glorified God,

LUKE 22:50-51 NKJ
50 And one of them struck the servant of the high priest and cut off his right ear.
51 But Jesus answered and said, "Permit even this." And He touched his ear and healed him.

JOHN 5:5-9 NKJ

5 Now a certain man was there who had an infirmity thirty-eight years.

6 When Jesus saw him lying there, and knew that he already had been in that condition a long time, He said to him, "Do you want to be made well?"

7 The sick man answered Him, "Sir, I have no man to put me into the pool when the water is stirred up; but while I am coming, another steps down before me."

8 Jesus said to him, "Rise, take up your bed and walk."

9 And immediately the man was made well, took up his bed, and walked. And that day was the Sabbath.

ACTS 9:33-34 NKJ

33 There he found a certain man named Aeneas, who had been bedridden eight years and was paralyzed.

34 And Peter said to him, "Aeneas, Jesus the Christ heals you. Arise and make your bed." Then he arose immediately.

Chapter 6

Scripture Confessions For Health

The personalized statements from God's Word on the following pages are full of God's power. They are God's medicine for you. So speak them often without becoming impatient. They will take root in you, change you, and bring forth a harvest of health.

SO SPEAK THEM ALOUD!

You are planting seeds of health and feeding your faith as you speak these words from the Bible.

Jesus is my Lord. God raised Him from the dead. He was my substitute. He is my Saviour; satan has no power over me. Jesus is my Lord. *(Philippians 2:11; Romans 10:9-10)*

I serve the One Whose Name is, "I Am the Lord Who heals you." *(Exodus 15:26)*

Jesus is the Healer; satan is the oppressor. For Acts 10:38 says "God anointed Jesus of Nazareth with the Holy Spirit and with power, Who went about doing good and healing all that were oppressed by the devil."

Jesus Christ is the same yesterday, and today, and forever. *(Hebrews 13:8)*

Jesus came that I may have life and have it in its fullness. *(John 10:10)*

God desires that I prosper and be in health. *(3 John 2)*

My God is supplying all I need according to His riches in glory by Christ Jesus. *(Philippians 4:19)*

The Lord is my Helper. I will not be afraid. *(Hebrews 13:6)*

God says in His Word in
Joel 3:10, "Let the weak
say, I am strong." I am
strong in the Lord.

God says in His Word
in Isaiah 33:24, "The
inhabitant will not say, I
am sick." Therefore I will
not say it. I will say what
God has said in His Word,
"By His wounds I have been
healed." *(1 Peter 2:24)*

Jesus says in Mark 11:23,
"whoever says to this
mountain, `Be removed,
and be cast into the sea,'
and does not doubt in
his heart, but believes

that those things he says will come to pass, he will have whatever he says." Therefore, mountain of sickness, be removed from me, and be cast into the sea. You have to because I command it in the authority of Jesus' Name.

According to Jesus, since I do not doubt in my heart, but I believe those things I say will come to pass, I will have what I say. Therefore, by faith, I will say these confessions.

Hebrews 3:1 and 4:14 say
Jesus is the High Priest of
my confession, so I will only
speak words that I desire
Jesus to say about me.

Death and life are in
the power of the tongue.
Therefore I will speak words
of life. Jesus says in John
6:63 that His words are
life, so I will speak them.
(Proverbs 18:21)

When I speak God's Word
I am planting good seed in
my life. *(Luke 8:11)*

I will hold fast to the
confession of God's Word
without wavering, for He

Who promised is faithful.
(Hebrews 10:23; Hebrews 4:14)

I do not waver at the promise of God through unbelief, but I am fully convinced that what He has promised He is also able to perform. *(Romans 4:20,21)*

I am not weak in faith, so I do not consider my own body above what God has said. *(Romans 4:19)*

I do not put my confidence in the flesh. *(Philippians 3:3)*

I'm not moved by what I feel. I'm not moved by what I see. For I "walk by faith, not by sight." *(2 Corinthians 5:7)* I'm moved only by what I believe. I believe the Word of God.

Father, your Word is truth. *(John 17:17)*

I will give attention to God's words, I will incline my ear to His sayings. I will not let them depart from my eyes. I will keep them in my heart. They are life to me for I have found them, and they are health, healing and medicine to all my flesh. *(Proverbs 4:20-22)*

Pleasant words are health, healing and medicine to my bones. *(Proverbs 16:24)*

God's Word of grace builds me up and gives me my inheritance. *(Acts 20:32)*

Jesus says if I continue in His Word, I will know the truth, and the truth will make me free. *(John 8:31-32)*

I have been called to freedom. *(Galatians 5:13)*

Because I am Christ's, I am a child of Abraham, and according to Jesus in Luke 13:16, I ought to be loosed from all bondage today (because God shows no partiality). *(Acts 10:34; Galatians 3:7,29)*

I am God's workmanship, created in Christ Jesus. *(Ephesians 2:10)*

I am a new creation in Christ Jesus. Old things have passed away. All things have become new and all things are of God. *(2 Corinthians 5:17)*

I am complete in Jesus, Who is the head of all rule and authority. *(Colossians 2:10)*

My body is the temple of the Holy Spirit Who is in me, and I am not my own. I am bought at a price. So I will glorify God in my body and my spirit. *(1 Corinthians 6:19-20)*

I present my body to God as a living sacrifice. *(Romans 12:1)*

Christ has redeemed me
from the curse of the law,
which includes all sickness.
So I forbid all sickness
and disease in my body.
Every disease germ and
virus that touches my body
dies instantly. Every cell,
organ, member, and system
of my body functions
perfectly, and I forbid
any malfunction, in the
supreme authority of the
Name of Jesus. *(Galatians 3:13;
Deuteronomy 28:61; Matthew 16:19;
Philippians 2:9)*

I am a believer. All things
are possible to me. *(Mark 9:23)*

I can do all things through Christ Who strengthens me. *(Philippians 4:13)*

The Lord is the strength of my life. *(Psalm 27:1)*

I am strong in the Lord and in His mighty power. *(Ephesians 6:10)*

Greater is He that is in me than he (the defeated one), that is in the world, (who is the author of sickness). *(1 John 4:4; Acts 10:38; Luke 13:16)*

My Father has made me able to be a partaker of my inheritance. He has delivered me from the authority of darkness, and has translated me into the kingdom of His dear Son, in Whom I have my redemption through His blood. *(Colossians 1:12-14)*

I am an overcomer and I overcome by the blood of the Lamb and the word of my testimony. *(1 John 4:4; Revelation 12:11)*

I am submitted to God by being submitted to His Word, and the devil flees from me because I resist him in the supreme authority of the Name of Jesus. *(James 4:7; Mark 16:17)*

No weapon formed against me shall prosper, for my righteousness is of the Lord. *(Isaiah 54:17; 1 Corinthians 1:30)*

There shall nothing evil happen to me, neither shall any plague or sickness come near me. *(Psalm 91:10)*

Jesus gave me authority over all the power of the enemy, and nothing shall hurt me. *(Luke 10:19; Mark 16:17)*

I do not return evil for evil, but on the contrary blessing, that I may obtain a blessing. *(1 Peter 3:9)*

I forgive others freely as God has forgiven me. I don't hold anything against anyone. *(Ephesians 4:32; Mark 11:25)*

I refrain my tongue from evil. I turn away from evil and do good. I seek peace and pursue it. So I will love life and see good days. *(1 Peter 3:10,11)*

I have a merry heart and that does me good like medicine. *(Proverbs 17:22)*

I have cast all my cares on the Lord for He cares for me. I refuse to worry about anything. *(1 Peter 5:7)*

I serve the Lord my God, and He blesses my bread, and my water, and He has taken sickness away from me. For Jesus, Himself, took my infirmities and bore my sicknesses away. *(Exodus 23:25; Matthew 8:17)*

Surely He has borne my
sicknesses and carried my
pains, yet we did esteem
Him stricken, smitten by
God, and afflicted. But
He was wounded for my
transgressions, He was
bruised for my iniquities,
the chastisement for my
peace was upon Him, and
by His stripes I am healed.
(Isaiah 53:4,5)

Christ my passover was
sacrificed for me. So all
sickness and death has
to pass over me and my
household. *(1 Corinthians 5:7;
Exodus 12)*

I am blessed above all people. The Lord has taken away from me all sickness. *(Deuteronomy 7:14,15)*

God sent His Word and healed me, and delivered me from destruction. *(Psalm 107:20)*

The number of my days God will fulfill. *(Exodus 23:26)*

Bless the Lord, O my soul; and all that is within me, bless His holy Name! Bless the Lord, O my soul, and forget not all His benefits: Who forgives all my iniquities, Who heals all my diseases, Who redeems my life from destruction, Who crowns me with lovingkindness and tender mercies, Who satisfies my mouth with good things, so that my youth is renewed like the eagle's. *(Psalm 103:1-5)*

JESUS LOVES ME!

Chapter 7

Questions

Why are some devout Christian believers sick?

No one can earn healing by serving God. Healing must be received as a gift, regardless of who you are. Sickness is an attack of the enemy, so we should not be surprised when Christian leaders are attacked.

Haven't there been people who received a miracle healing, yet had no faith?

This happens occasionally, just as we occasionally hear of an angel telling someone how to find forgiveness in Christ. But it would be foolish for someone to wait on an angelic appearance when God's Word already explains the plan of salvation through Jesus Christ.

Only God knows all the reasons things happen to some people. (Probably someone was praying for them.) We don't know everything. But we can know what God has plainly told us in the Bible, and we can believe it.

People can also be healed, re-gardless of their faith for healing, through the faith of the person min-istering to them. This book does not focus on this way of receiving healing.

Are you saying God's will is healing, every time, for every person?
Yes! Ideally, that's true. But, just as it is God's will for all to come to

the knowledge of the truth and believe in Jesus Christ, not everyone
does. What we believe determines
what we will experience.

As we release faith in what Jesus
has done, a process of healing be-
gins. Then, as we stay in faith and
continue to feed on God's Word,
our thinking, talking, and acting
will change as God works in us —
resulting in health.

Healing is always God's best will for
ALL of us, not just a selected few.

**Doesn't human experience show
that healing is not God's will for
everyone?**
We cannot judge God's will by what
people do. To determine God's
will, we should examine what God
Himself has plainly said. Just because some people in the past
have not clearly understood and

embraced God's provision for their healing, is not a good reason for you to suffer.

Jesus loves you and yearns for you to receive all that He paid for you to enjoy. Don't allow unbelief to rob you!

> MATTHEW 13:58 NKJ
> 58 Now He did not do many mighty works there because of their unbelief.

> HEBREWS 3:19 NKJ
> 19 So we see that they could not enter in because of unbelief.

Why are some not healed?

Why do some people not accept the salvation and forgiveness offered by Jesus Christ? Jesus died for all. But not all believe, and actively accept what Jesus did for them. The main reason people are not healed

is simply because they have never
been told healing is available for
them. Others have not received
healing because no one explained
to them how to receive in a way they
could understand. So, through ignorance, the devil robs them of
what Jesus paid for them to enjoy.

**Are you condemning people for
not having faith to be healed?**
NO! The spirit of Jesus is not to
condemn people. He came to help
us. Jesus does not reveal truth to
condemn us, but only to free us.
Being offended by revealed truth is
a mistake that robs us of blessings.

The reason people don't have faith
is simply because they have not
heard the truth clearly. Faith is
not something you are born with.
People lack faith in Jesus providing
for their healing mainly because no
one has ever told them. That's why

you need the message of this book, taken directly from Scripture.

I have compassion for all people who hurt, and in no way want to condemn anyone. My desire is to clearly communicate that God loves you right now, just as you are. And God has already made provision for you to be healed.

But I know someone who had great faith, yet was not healed.
A major problem has been thinking that all healing must be instantaneous. People can be healed, or at least start the healing process, but then decide to abandon their faith.

God does His part, but if we don't actively receive our healing, the devil can steal it from us through doubt. Not understanding that God's healing is a process involving time has certainly been a problem.

MATTHEW 13:19 NKJ
19 "When anyone hears the word of the kingdom, and does not understand it, then the wicked one comes and snatches away what was sown in his heart. This is he who received seed by the wayside.

You need to understand that someone can have great faith in God, but still not believe it is God's will to heal them. Many have been taught human tradition about healing instead of clear Scriptural truth.

No one but God knows what any person truly believes. So trying to determine God's will by what other people receive is a foolish approach.

I do not judge people or condemn anyone, but encourage you to receive all that Jesus paid for you to have, and to remind you how much

God loves you — even if you don't believe His Word.

This book just shows you what God said in the Bible. When you choose to believe what God said, the healing process will begin in your body.

But wasn't all healing during Jesus' ministry on earth instantaneous?

Not always. Mark 8:22-25 is an account of Jesus ministering to a blind man. After Jesus laid hands on the blind man he could "see men like trees, walking."

In other words, he could see, but not very well. Only when Jesus laid hands on him again did his sight become clear. Although a long period of time was not involved, it does show a healing that was a process — not instantaneous.

> MARK 8:25 NKJ
> 25 Then He put His hands on
> his eyes again and made him
> look up. And he was restored
> and saw everyone clearly.

Luke 17:12-19 tells of ten lepers who were healed "as they went."

Healing was not manifest while they were in Jesus' presence, but only after they left Him.

> LUKE 17:14 NKJ
> 14 So when He saw them, He
> said to them, "Go, show your-
> selves to the priests." And so
> it was that as they went, they
> were cleansed.

John 9:6-7 tells of another healing involving the passage of some time.

As our faith grows stronger, we will probably see the healing process speed up most of the time.

Why do some people receive healing, then get sick again?

We live in a fallen world, and sickness is a fact we have to deal with. Scripture reveals that sickness is an attack from our enemy. So we must learn to resist sickness. And we should not be surprised to experience more than one attack.

Instead of waiting until sickness has a firm hold in our life, at the first symptom of any sickness we should command it to leave us, and stand our ground in faith on God's Word.

Jesus resisted satan's attacks by speaking the written Word of God. We must do the same.

Jesus loves us just as much regardless of how we respond, but it gives Him no pleasure to see us suffer needlessly.

We need to choose to actively resist all that is from the devil, and actively receive all that is from God. Jesus does not force any blessing on us. We must submit to God and resist the devil, which means resisting all his works — including sickness.

What do you mean by saying sickness is an attack from our enemy?

I certainly do not mean the devil is personally present, or directly causing every sickness. But Scripture reveals that sickness originated as a result of Adam listening to satan and rebelling against God. So the devil is ultimately behind all sickness, which is death in its beginning stages.

> ROMANS 5:12 NLT
> 12 When Adam sinned, sin entered the world. Adam's sin

brought death, so death spread to everyone, for everyone sinned.

Verses such as Acts 10:38 and Luke 13:16 show that Jesus and His disciples blamed sickness on the devil. Jesus, our example (John 14:12), spoke directly to sickness in the same way He spoke to demons (Mark 9:25, Luke 4:35, 39).

Why are some people healed quickly, while others take a long time to completely recover?

Only God, who makes every fingerprint unique, can fully answer this question. People are individuals.

But God is working out His best will for every one of us as we submit to Him. We can trust in His perfect love. Our part is to simply believe His Word and be grateful for what God has given us — not to complain about what someone else got.

Instead of expressing doubt or unbelief if healing does not happen quickly, we should respond by saying "Thank You Lord that Your healing power is working in my body now!"

Are you saying that people who are sick deserve to be sick?

NO! Some sickness may be a result of unhealthy lifestyle choices we have made, but certainly not always. Many people are victims of accidents and the bad choices of others. No one deserves to be sick.

Their bad choices may have made an opening for sickness to attack them. But Jesus died for all our sins. God forgives, so we should also forgive ourselves as well as others. We all need God's mercy.

Must I be perfect to receive healing from God?

NO! If only perfect people received help from God, none of us would ever receive anything! All of us have fallen short and need God's grace. Receiving healing from God is not a struggle, it's a free gift available to all!

Why doesn't Jesus just force everyone to be healed?

He gave us the freedom to choose — to accept Him and His blessings — or to reject Him. Love does not force others. Love invites. The Bible shows us that God loves us with a perfect love.

But isn't suffering God's way of perfecting us?

NO! Illness has never made anyone a better person. How a person chooses to respond to suffering makes the difference.

Some people experience great suffering and become better people because they turn to God in their suffering, and receive His grace to change.

But many people become worse because of suffering. So, we should never credit suffering for improving people, but credit God. Sickness is one kind of suffering a Christian should be freed from, because Jesus redeemed us from sickness.

What about all the bad pollution in the world: chemicals and toxins that make us sick?

We should endeavor to live a healthy lifestyle and take care of the bodies God has given us. We cannot avoid all the bad in the world, but God's power is certainly able to overcome its effects. No matter what has caused your sickness, the power of God is sufficient to cure it.

Does this mean I can just read the healing Scriptures each day and continue my unhealthy lifestyle and still expect to stay healthy?

When people are in a situation they have no control over, God seems to supply extra grace to compensate. But when people know what is right, but refuse to do what they know they should do, the results are usually not good.

While we cannot "earn" our healing by keeping any list of rules, no one should be deceived into thinking they can ignore God's instruction and continue to avoid any bad consequences.

Jesus paid for us all to be healed. But if we rebel against God and refuse to heed His instruction, we are choosing to reject God's gracious gifts. While His healing power may come every time, by refusing to listen to God, we also open the door for sickness to come back on us.

God's medicine is meant to change your thinking — so you will think, talk, and act in line with what God says in His Word. (Even medical science has proven that our thoughts and our words affect our physical bodies.) A primary way God's medicine works is by changing us.

Why doesn't my church teach this?

A prevalent idea is: "If our group doesn't teach it, then it can't be true." This can be a deadly mistake. We all have much to learn. Even the Apostle Paul, who was taught directly by Jesus Himself, said he only knew in part.

The devil has robbed Christians because we have not clearly

understood healing. Your teachers and church leaders are probably compassionate and well-meaning individuals. But people generally just teach what they were taught. If their teachers did not understand about healing, it's unrealistic to expect they will either.

How will we die, if we are not sick?

Many people in the Bible died without sickness. All you have to do to die is quit breathing.

But no matter how you die, as a believer in Jesus Christ, you can know you are headed to Heaven to be with Jesus for all eternity — and He will receive you with love, acceptance, and forgiveness.

What a wonderful hope Jesus has given us because of His great love for us!

Afterword

God has *already* made provision for your healing. But you must actively receive that provision by faith. Faith believes what God says, regardless of circumstances or feelings.

Actively receiving means "Take it!" Lay claim to it and consider it your own. Then be ready to resist any attempt to steal it away from you.

Your faith will grow as you boldly and consistently say the statements from God's Word in this book. As you continue to meditate on and boldly speak God's Word, it will produce healing and wholeness in your life. It works just like a seed bringing forth a harvest.

God will surely perform His Word.

JEREMIAH 1:12 NIV
12 The LORD said to me, "You have seen correctly, for I am watching to see that my word is fulfilled."

This book is not to read just once and lay aside. Use it regularly as food for your faith, even when you are healthy. You cannot overdose on God's medicine, which is also effective for disease prevention.

This marvelous medicine deserves to be shared. Everyone you love should have a copy of this book readily available when they need it.

May our wonderful Lord Jesus Christ be forever praised and thanked for all He has done for us!

There is no sickness in Heaven. *May God's will be done on Earth as it is in Heaven!* (Matthew 6:10)

Ordering Information

This book may be purchased at www.amazon.com. Additional ordering information is available at: www.CFApublications.com where you can also obtain a free online copy.

Every home should have this book on hand, making it easy to access God's medicine. Consider giving one to all your family and friends.

If you were helped by this book, please consider leaving your comments at www.amazon.com so others will be encouraged to read it too.

Audio of the Scripture Confessions For Health starting on page 127 may be downloaded free of charge from www.believers.org/healing/